CW00495084

Diabetic Cookbook

Easy Lean and Green Recipes to Quickly Start Weight Loss for Beginners, easy and healthy diabetic recipes to improve nutrition

TABLE OF CONTENTS

—

3

The information in the following pages is broadly considered a truthful and accurate account of facts and as such, any inattention, use, or misuse of the information in question by the reader will render any resulting actions solely under their purview. There are no scenarios in which the publisher or the original author of this work can be in any fashion deemed liable for any hardship or damages that may befall them after undertaking information described herein.

Additionally, the information in the following pages is intended only for informational purposes and should thus be thought of as universal. As befitting its nature, it is presented without assurance regarding its prolonged validity or interim quality. Trademarks that are mentioned are done without written consent and can in no way be considered an endorsement from the trademark holder.

Chocolate Quinoa Brownies

Preparation Time: 10 minutes

Cooking time: 2 hours

Servings: 16

Ingredients

- 2 eggs
- 3 cups quinoa, cooked
- 1 teaspoon vanilla liquid stevia
- 1 ¼ chocolate chips, sugar free
- 1 teaspoon vanilla extract
- 1/3 cup flaxseed ground
- ¼ teaspoon salt
- 1/3 cup cocoa powder, unsweetened
- 1/2 teaspoon baking powder
- 1 teaspoon pure stevia extract
- 1/2 cup applesauce, unsweetened

Sugar- frees frosting:

- ¼ cup heavy cream
- 1 teaspoon chocolate liquid stevia
- ¼ cup cocoa powder, unsweetened
- 1/2 teaspoon vanilla extract

DIRECTIONS:

1. Add all the ingredients to a food processor. Then process until well incorporated.

2. Line a crock pot with a parchment paper, and then spread the batter into the lined pot.

3. Close the lid and cook for 4 hours on LOW or 2 hours on HIGH. Let cool.

4. Prepare the frosting. Whisk all the ingredients together and then microwave for 20 seconds. Taste and adjust on sweetener if desired.

5. When the frosting is ready, stir it well again and then pour it over the sliced brownies.

6. Serve and enjoy!

Nutrition: 133 calories; 7.9 g fat; 18.4 g total carbs; 4.3 g protein

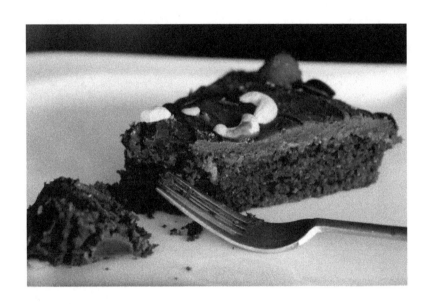

Blueberry Crisp

Preparation Time: 10 minutes

Cooking time: 3-4 hours

Servings: 10

Ingredients

- 1/4 cup butter, melted

- 24 oz. blueberries, frozen

- 3/4 teaspoon salt

- 1 1/2 cups rolled oats, coarsely ground

- 3/4 cup almond flour, blanched

- 1/4 cup coconut oil, melted

- 6 tablespoons sweetener

- 1 cup pecans or walnuts, coarsely chopped

Directions:

1. Using a non-stick cooking spray, spray the slow cooker pot well.

2. Into a bowl, add ground oats and chopped nuts along with salt, blanched almond flour, brown sugar, stevia granulated sweetener, and then stir in the coconut/butter mixture. Stir well to combine.

3. When done, spread crisp topping over blueberries. Cook for 3-4 hours, until the mixture has become bubbling hot and you can smell the blueberries.

4. Serve while still hot with the whipped cream or the ice cream if desired. Enjoy!

Nutrition: 261 calories; 16.6 g fat; 32 g total carbs; 4 g protein

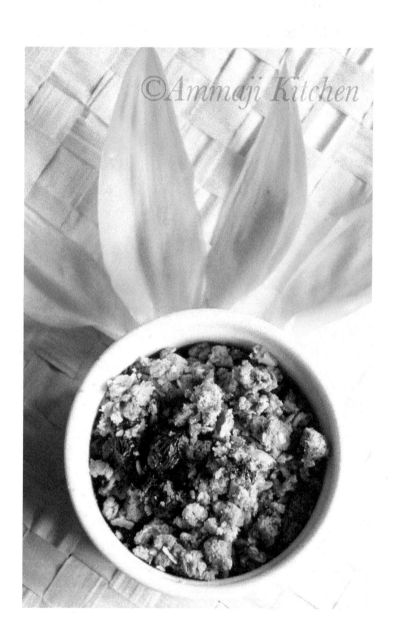

Maple Custard

Preparation Time: 10 minutes

Cooking time: 2 hours

Servings: 6

Ingredients

- 1 teaspoon maple extract

- 2 egg yolks

- 1 cup heavy cream

- 2 eggs

- 1/2 cup whole milk

- 1/4 teaspoon salt

- 1/4 cup Sukrin Gold or any sugar-free brown sugar substitute

- 1/2 teaspoon cinnamon

Directions:

1. Combine all ingredients together in a blender, process well.

2. Grease 6 ramekins and then pour the batter evenly into each ramekin.

3. To the bottom of the slow cooker, add 4 ramekins and then arrange the remaining 2 against the side of a slow cooker, and not at the top of bottom ramekins.

4. Close the lid and cook on high for 2 hours, until the center is cooked through but the middle is still jiggly.

5. Let cool at a room temperature for an hour after removing from the slow cooker, and then chill in the fridge for at least 2 hours.

6. Serve and enjoy with a sprinkle of cinnamon and little sugar free whipped cream.

Nutrition: 190 calories; 18 g fat; 2 g total carbs; 4 g protein

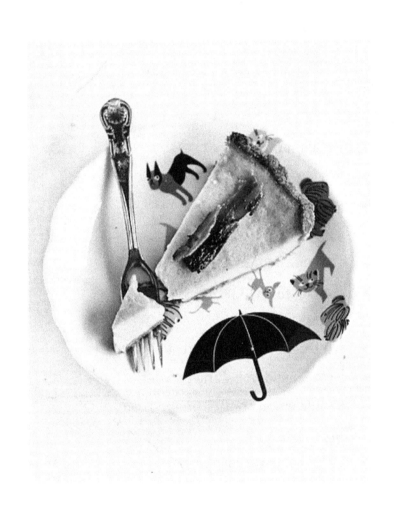

Raspberry Cream Cheese Coffee Cake

Preparation Time: 10 minutes

Cooking time: 4 hours

Servings: 12

Ingredients

- 1 1/4 almond flour
- 2/3 cup water
- 1/2 cup Swerve
- 3 eggs
- 1/4 cup coconut flour
- 1/4 cup protein powder
- 1/4 teaspoon salt
- 1/2 teaspoon vanilla extract
- 1 1/2 teaspoon baking powder
- 6 tablespoons butter, melted

For the Filling:

- 1 1/2 cup fresh raspberries
- 8 oz. cream cheese
- 1 large egg
- 1/3 cup powdered Swerve
- 2 tablespoon whipping cream

DIRECTIONS:

1. Grease the slow cooker pot. Prepare the cake batter. In a bowl, combine almond flour together with coconut flour, sweetener, baking powder, protein powder and salt, and then stir in the melted butter along with eggs and water until well combined. Set aside.

2. Prepare the filling. Beat cream cheese thoroughly with the sweetener until have smoothened, and then beat in whipping cream along with the egg and vanilla extract until well combined.

3. Assemble the cake. Spread around 2/3 of batter in the slow cooker as you smoothen the top using a spatula or knife.

4. Pour cream cheese mixture over the batter in the pan, evenly spread it, and then sprinkle with raspberries. Add the rest of batter over filling.

5. Cook for 3-4 hours on low. Let cool completely.

6. Serve and enjoy!

Nutrition: 239 calories; 19.18 g fat; 6.9 g total carbs; 7.5 g protein

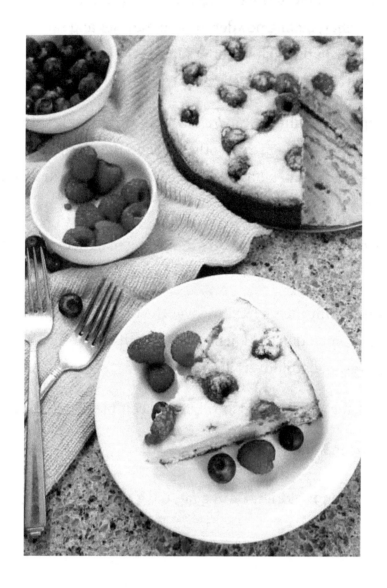

Pumpkin Pie Bars

Preparation Time: 10 minutes

Cooking time: 3 hours

Servings: 16

Ingredients

For the Crust:

- 3/4 cup coconut, shredded
- 4 tablespoons butter, unsalted, softened
- 1/4 cup cocoa powder, unsweetened
- 1/4 teaspoon salt
- 1/2 cup raw sunflower seeds or sunflower seed flour
- 1/4 cup confectioners Swerve

Filling:

- 2 teaspoons cinnamon liquid stevia
- 1 cup heavy cream
- 1 can pumpkin puree
- 6 eggs
- 1 tablespoon pumpkin pie spice
- 1/2 teaspoon salt
- 1 tablespoon vanilla extract
- 1/2 cup sugar-free chocolate chips, optional

Directions:

1. Add all the crust ingredients to a food processor. Then process until fine crumbs are formed.

2. Grease the slow cooker pan well. When done, press crust mixture onto the greased bottom.

3. In a stand mixer, combine all the ingredients for the filling, and then blend well until combined.

4. Top the filling with chocolate chips if using, and then pour the mixture onto the prepared crust.

5. Close the lid and cook for 3 hours on low. Open the lid and let cool for at least 30 minutes, and then place the slow cooker into the refrigerator for at least 3 hours.

6. Slice the pumpkin pie bar and serve it with sugar free whipped cream. Enjoy!

Nutrition: 169 calories; 15 g fat; 6 g total carbs; 4 g protein

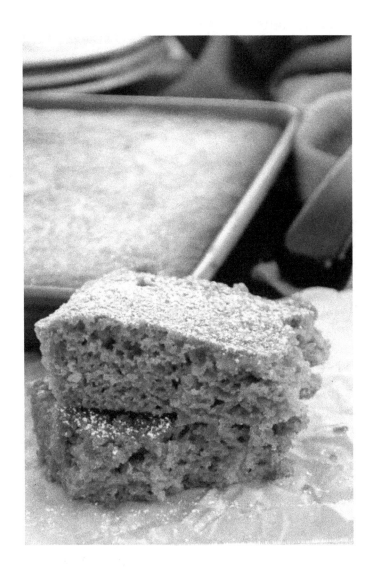

Dark Chocolate Cake

Preparation Time: 10 minutes

Cooking time: 3 hours

Servings: 10

Ingredients

- 1 cup almond flour

- 3 eggs

- 2 tablespoons almond flour

- 1/4 teaspoon salt

- 1/2 cup Swerve Granular

- 3/4 teaspoon vanilla extract

- 2/3 cup almond milk, unsweetened

- 1/2 cup cocoa powder

- 6 tablespoons butter, melted

- 1 1/2 teaspoon baking powder

- 3 tablespoon unflavored whey protein powder or egg white protein powder

- 1/3 cup sugar-free chocolate chips, optional

Directions:

1. Grease the slow cooker well.

2. Whisk the almond flour together with cocoa powder, sweetener, whey protein powder, salt and baking powder in a bowl. Then stir in butter along with almond milk, eggs and the vanilla extract until well combined, and then stir in the chocolate chips if desired.

3. When done, pour into the slow cooker. Allow to cook for 2-2 1/2 hours on low.

4. When through, turn off the slow cooker and let the cake cool for about 20-30 minutes.

5. When cooled, cut the cake into pieces and serve warm with lightly sweetened whipped cream. Enjoy!

Nutrition: 205 calories; 17 g fat; 8.4 g total carbs; 12 g protein

Lemon Custard

Preparation Time: 10 minutes

Cooking time: 3 hours

Servings: 4

Ingredients:

- 2 cups whipping cream or coconut cream

- 5 egg yolks

- 1 tablespoon lemon zest

- 1 teaspoon vanilla extract

- 1/4 cup fresh lemon juice, squeezed

- 1/2 teaspoon liquid stevia

- Lightly sweetened whipped cream

Directions:

1. Whisk egg yolks together with lemon zest, liquid stevia, lemon zest and vanilla in a bowl, and then whisk in heavy cream.

2. Divide the mixture among 4 small jars or ramekins.

3. To the bottom of a slow cooker add a rack, and then add ramekins on top of the rack and add enough water to cover half of ramekins.

4. Close the lid and cook for 3 hours on low. Remove ramekins.

5. Let cool to room temperature, and then place into the refrigerator to cool completely for about 3 hours.

6. When through, top with the whipped cream and serve. Enjoy!

Nutrition: 319 calories; 30 g fat; 3 g total carbs; 7 g protein

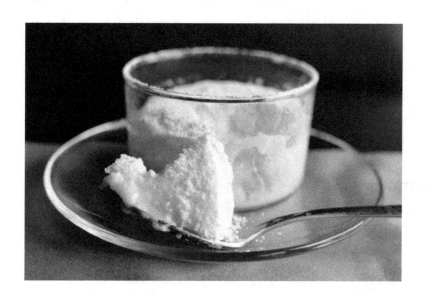

Pumpkin & Banana Ice Cream

Preparation Time: 5 minutes

Cooking Time: 10 minutes

Servings: 4

Ingredients:

- 15 oz. pumpkin puree

- 4 bananas, sliced and frozen

- 1 teaspoon pumpkin pie spice

- Chopped pecans

Directions:

1.Add pumpkin puree, bananas and pumpkin pie spice in a food processor.

2.Pulse until smooth.

3.Chill in the refrigerator.

4.Garnish with pecans.

Nutrition:

71 Calories

18g Carbohydrate

1.2g Protein

Brulee Oranges

Preparation Time: 5 minutes

Cooking Time: 10 minutes

Servings: 4

Ingredients:

- 4 oranges, sliced into segments

- 1 teaspoon ground cardamom

- 6 teaspoons brown sugar

- 1 cup nonfat Greek yogurt

Directions:

1.Preheat your broiler.

2.Arrange orange slices in a baking pan.

3.In a bowl, mix the cardamom and sugar.

4.Sprinkle mixture on top of the oranges. Broil for 5 minutes.

5.Serve oranges with yogurt.

Nutrition:

168 Calories

26.9g Carbohydrate

6.8g Protein

Frozen Lemon & Blueberry

Preparation Time: 5 minutes

Cooking Time: 10 minutes

Servings: 4

Ingredients:

- 6 cup fresh blueberries

- 8 sprigs fresh thyme

- ¾ cup light brown sugar

- 1 teaspoon lemon zest

- ¼ cup lemon juice

- 2 cups water

Directions:

1.Add blueberries, thyme and sugar in a pan over medium heat.

2.Cook for 6 to 8 minutes.

3.Transfer mixture to a blender.

4.Remove thyme sprigs.

5.Stir in the remaining ingredients.

6.Pulse until smooth.

7.Strain mixture and freeze for 1 hour.

Nutrition:

78 Calories

20g Carbohydrate

3g Protein

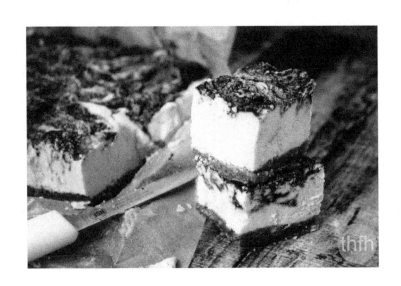

Peanut Butter Choco Chip Cookies

Preparation Time: 5 minutes

Cooking Time: 10 minutes

Servings: 4

Ingredients:

- 1 egg

- ½ cup light brown sugar

- 1 cup natural unsweetened peanut butter

- Pinch salt

- ¼ cup dark chocolate chips

Directions:

1.Preheat your oven to 375 degrees F.

2.Mix egg, sugar, peanut butter, salt and chocolate chips in a bowl.

3.Form into cookies and place in a baking pan.

4.Bake the cookie for 10 minutes.

5.Let cool before serving.

Nutrition:

159 Calories

12g Carbohydrate

4.3g Protein

Watermelon Sherbet

Preparation Time: 5 minutes

Cooking Time: 3 minutes

Servings: 4

Ingredients:

- 6 cups watermelon, sliced into cubes

- 14 oz. almond milk

- 1 tablespoon honey

- ¼ cup lime juice

- Salt to taste

Directions:

1. Freeze watermelon for 4 hours.

2. Add frozen watermelon and other ingredients in a blender.

3. Blend until smooth.

4. Transfer to a container with seal.

5. Seal and freeze for 4 hours.

Nutrition:

132 Calories

24.5g Carbohydrate

3.1g Protein

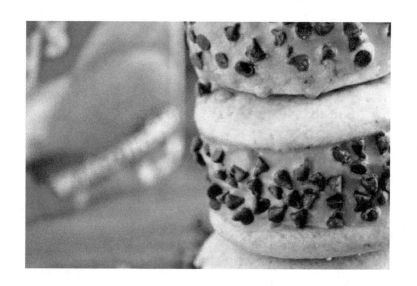

Strawberry & Mango Ice Cream

Preparation Time: 5 minutes

Cooking Time: 10 minutes

Servings: 4

Ingredients:

- 8 oz. strawberries, sliced

- 12 oz. mango, sliced into cubes

- 1 tablespoon lime juice

Directions:

1.Add all ingredients in a food processor.

2.Pulse for 2 minutes.

3.Chill before serving.

Nutrition:

70 Calories

17.4g Carbohydrate

1.1g Protein

Sparkling Fruit Drink

Preparation Time: 5 minutes

Cooking Time: 10 minutes

Servings: 4

Ingredients:

- 8 oz. unsweetened grape juice

- 8 oz. unsweetened apple juice

- 8 oz. unsweetened orange juice

- 1 qt. homemade ginger ale

- Ice

Directions:

1.Makes 7 servings. Mix first 4 ingredients together in a pitcher. Stir in ice cubes and 9 ounces of the beverage to each glass. Serve immediately.

Nutrition:

60 Calories

1.1g Protein

Tiramisu Shots

Preparation Time: 5 minutes

Cooking Time: 10 minutes

Servings: 4

Ingredients:

- 1 pack silken tofu

- 1 oz. dark chocolate, finely chopped

- ¼ cup sugar substitute

- 1 teaspoon lemon juice

- ¼ cup brewed espresso

- Pinch salt

- 24 slices angel food cake

- Cocoa powder (unsweetened)

Directions:

1.Add tofu, chocolate, sugar substitute, lemon juice, espresso and salt in a food processor.

2.Pulse until smooth.

3.Add angel food cake pieces into shot glasses.

4.Drizzle with the cocoa powder.

5.Pour the tofu mixture on top.

6.Top with the remaining angel food cake pieces.

7.Chill for 30 minutes and serve.

Nutrition:

75 Calories

12g Carbohydrate

2.9g Protein

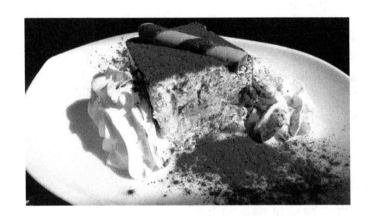

Ice Cream Brownie Cake

Preparation Time: 5 minutes

Cooking Time: 10 minutes

Servings: 4

Ingredients:

- Cooking spray

- 12 oz. no-sugar brownie mix

- ¼ cup oil

- 2 egg whites

- 3 tablespoons water

- 2 cups sugar-free ice cream

Directions:

1. Preheat your oven to 325 degrees F.

2. Spray your baking pan with oil.

3. Mix brownie mix, oil, egg whites and water in a bowl.

4. Pour into the baking pan.

5. Bake for 25 minutes.

6. Let cool.

7. Freeze brownie for 2 hours.

8. Spread ice cream over the brownie.

9. Freeze for 8 hours.

Nutrition:

198 Calories

33g Carbohydrate

3g Protein

Peanut Butter Cups

Preparation Time: 5 minutes

Cooking Time: 10 minutes

Servings: 4

Ingredients:

- 1 packet plain gelatin

- ¼ cup sugar substitute

- 2 cups nonfat cream

- ½ teaspoon vanilla

- ¼ cup low-fat peanut butter

- 2 tablespoons unsalted peanuts, chopped

Directions:

1.Mix gelatin, sugar substitute and cream in a pan.

2.Let sit for 5 minutes.

3.Place over medium heat and cook until gelatin has been dissolved.

4.Stir in vanilla and peanut butter.

5.Pour into custard cups. Chill for 3 hours.

6.Top with the peanuts and serve.

Nutrition:

171 Calories

21g Carbohydrate

6.8g Protein

Fruit Pizza

Preparation Time: 5 minutes

Cooking Time: 10 minutes

Servings: 4

Ingredients:

- 1 teaspoon maple syrup

- ¼ teaspoon vanilla extract

- ½ cup coconut milk yogurt

- 2 round slices watermelon

- ½ cup blackberries, sliced

- ½ cup strawberries, sliced

- 2 tablespoons coconut flakes (unsweetened)

Directions:

1.Mix maple syrup, vanilla and yogurt in a bowl.

2.Spread the mixture on top of the watermelon slice.

3.Top with the berries and coconut flakes.

Nutrition:

70 Calories

14.6g Carbohydrate

1.2g Protein

Choco Peppermint Cake

Preparation Time: 5 minutes

Cooking Time: 10 minutes

Servings: 4

Ingredients:

- Cooking spray

- 1/3 cup oil

- 15 oz. package chocolate cake mix

- 3 eggs, beaten

- 1 cup water

- ¼ teaspoon peppermint extract

Directions:

1.Spray slow cooker with oil.

2.Mix all the ingredients in a bowl.

3.Use an electric mixer on medium speed setting to mix ingredients for 2 minutes.

4.Pour mixture into the slow cooker.

5.Cover the pot and cook on low for 3 hours.

6.Let cool before slicing and serving.

Nutrition:

185 Calories

27g Carbohydrate

3.8g Protein

Roasted Mango

Preparation Time: 5 minutes

Cooking Time: 10 minutes

Servings: 4

Ingredients:

- 2 mangoes, sliced

- 2 teaspoons crystallized ginger, chopped

- 2 teaspoons orange zest

- 2 tablespoons coconut flakes (unsweetened)

Directions:

1.Preheat your oven to 350 degrees F.

2.Add mango slices in custard cups.

3.Top with the ginger, orange zest and coconut flakes.

4.Bake in the oven for 10 minutes.

Nutrition:

89 Calories

20g Carbohydrate

0.8g Protein

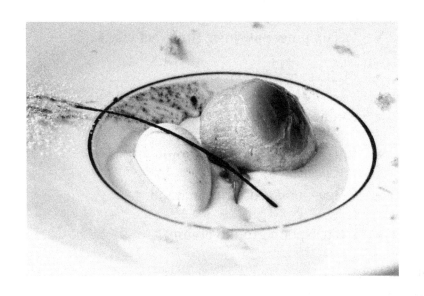

Roasted Plums

Preparation Time: 5 minutes

Cooking Time: 10 minutes

Servings: 4

Ingredients:

- Cooking spray

- 6 plums, sliced

- ½ cup pineapple juice (unsweetened)

- 1 tablespoon brown sugar

- 2 tablespoons brown sugar

- ¼ teaspoon ground cardamom

- ½ teaspoon ground cinnamon

- 1/8 teaspoon ground cumin

Directions:

1.Combine all the ingredients in a baking pan.

2.Roast in the oven at 450 degrees F for 20 minutes.

Nutrition:

102 Calories

18.7g Carbohydrate

2g Protein

Figs with Honey & Yogurt

Preparation Time: 5 minutes

Cooking Time: 10 minutes

Servings: 4

Ingredients:

- ½ teaspoon vanilla

- 8 oz. nonfat yogurt

- 2 figs, sliced

- 1 tablespoon walnuts, chopped and toasted

- 2 teaspoons honey

Directions:

1.Stir vanilla into yogurt.

2.Mix well.

3.Top with the figs and sprinkle with walnuts.

4.Drizzle with honey and serve.

Nutrition:

157 Calories

24g Carbohydrate

7g Protein

Flourless Chocolate Cake

Preparation Time: 10 minutes

Cooking Time: 45 minutes

Servings: 6

Ingredients:

- ½ Cup of stevia

- 12 Ounces of unsweetened baking chocolate

- 2/3 Cup of ghee

- 1/3 Cup of warm water

- ¼ Teaspoon of salt

- 4 Large pastured eggs

- 2 Cups of boiling water

Directions:

1.Line the bottom of a 9-inch pan of a spring form with a parchment paper.

2.Heat the water in a small pot; then add the salt and the stevia over the water until wait until the mixture becomes completely dissolved.

3.Melt the baking chocolate into a double boiler or simply microwave it for about 30 seconds.

4.Mix the melted chocolate and the butter in a large bowl with an electric mixer.

5.Beat in your hot mixture; then crack in the egg and whisk after adding each of the eggs.

6.Pour the obtained mixture into your prepared spring form tray.

7.Wrap the spring form tray with a foil paper.

8.Place the spring form tray in a large cake tray and add boiling water right to the outside; make sure the depth doesn't exceed 1 inch.

9.Bake the cake into the water bath for about 45 minutes at a temperature of about 350 F.

10.Remove the tray from the boiling water and transfer to a wire to cool.

11.Let the cake chill for an overnight in the refrigerator.

Nutrition

295 Calories

6g Carbohydrates

4g Fiber

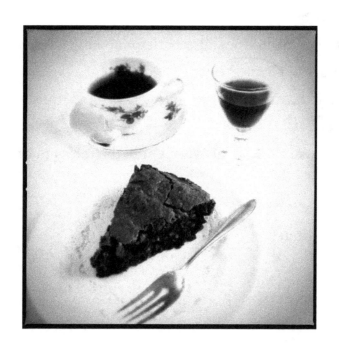

Raspberry Cake with White Chocolate Sauce

Preparation Time: 15 minutes

Cooking Time: 60 minutes

Servings: 5

Ingredients:

- 5 Ounces of melted cacao butter

- 2 Ounces of grass-fed ghee

- ½ Cup of coconut cream

- 1 Cup of green banana flour

- 3 Teaspoons of pure vanilla

- 4 Large eggs

- ½ Cup of as Lakanto Monk Fruit

- 1 Teaspoon of baking powder

- 2 Teaspoons of apple cider vinegar

- 2 Cup of raspberries

For white chocolate sauce:

- 3 and ½ ounces of cacao butter

- ½ Cup of coconut cream

- 2 Teaspoons of pure vanilla extract

- 1 Pinch of salt

Directions:

1.Preheat your oven to a temperature of about 280 degrees Fahrenheit.

2.Combine the green banana flour with the pure vanilla extract, the baking powder, the coconut cream, the eggs, the cider vinegar and the monk fruit and mix very well.

3.Leave the raspberries aside and line a cake loaf tin with a baking paper.

4.Pour in the batter into the baking tray and scatter the raspberries over the top of the cake.

5.Place the tray in your oven and bake it for about 60 minutes; in the meantime, prepare the sauce by

Directions for sauce:

6.Combine the cacao cream, the vanilla extract, the cacao butter and the salt in a saucepan over a low heat.

7.Mix all your ingredients with a fork to make sure the cacao butter mixes very well with the cream.

8.Remove from the heat and set aside to cool a little bit; but don't let it harden.

9.Drizzle with the chocolate sauce.

10.Scatter the cake with more raspberries.

11.Slice your cake; then serve and enjoy it!

Nutrition

323 Calories

9.9g Carbohydrates

4g Fiber

Lava Cake

Preparation Time: 10 minutes

Cooking Time: 10 minutes

Servings: 2

Ingredients:

- 2 Oz of dark chocolate; you should at least use chocolate of 85% cocoa solids

- 1 Tablespoon of super-fine almond flour

- 2 Oz of unsalted almond butter

- 2 Large eggs

Directions:

1.Heat your oven to a temperature of about 350 Fahrenheit.

2.Grease 2 heat proof ramekins with almond butter.

3.Now, melt the chocolate and the almond butter and stir very well.

4.Beat the eggs very well with a mixer.

5.Add the eggs to the chocolate and the butter mixture and mix very well with almond flour and the swerve; then stir.

6.Pour the dough into 2 ramekins.

7.Bake for about 9 to 10 minutes.

8.Turn the cakes over plates and serve with pomegranate seeds!

Nutrition

459 Calories

3.5g Carbohydrates

0.8g Fiber

Cheese Cake

Preparation Time: 15 minutes

Cooking Time: 50 minutes

Servings: 6

Ingredients:

For Almond Flour Cheesecake Crust:

- 2 Cups of Blanched almond flour

- 1/3 Cup of almond Butter

- 3 Tablespoons of Erythritol (powdered or granular)

- 1 Teaspoon of Vanilla extract

For Keto Cheesecake Filling:

- 32 Oz of softened Cream cheese

- 1 and ¼ cups of powdered erythritol

- 3 Large Eggs

- 1 Tablespoon of Lemon juice

- 1 Teaspoon of Vanilla extract

Directions:

1.Preheat your oven to a temperature of about 350 degrees F.

2.Grease a spring form pan of 9¨ with cooking spray or just line its bottom with a parchment paper.

3.In order to make the cheesecake rust, stir in the melted butter, the almond flour, the vanilla extract and the erythritol in a large bowl.

4.The dough will get will be a bit crumbly; so, press it into the bottom of your prepared tray.

5.Bake for about 12 minutes; then let cool for about 10 minutes.

6.In the meantime, beat the softened cream cheese and the powdered sweetener at a low speed until it becomes smooth.

7.Crack in the eggs and beat them in at a low to medium speed until it becomes fluffy. Make sure to add one a time.

8.Add in the lemon juice and the vanilla extract and mix at a low to medium speed with a mixer.

9.Pour your filling into your pan right on top of the crust. You can use a spatula to smooth the top of the cake.

10.Bake for about 45 to 50 minutes.

11.Remove the baked cheesecake from your oven and run a knife around its edge.

12.Let the cake cool for about 4 hours in the refrigerator.

13.Serve and enjoy your delicious cheese cake!

Nutrition

325 Calories

6g Carbohydrates

1g Fiber

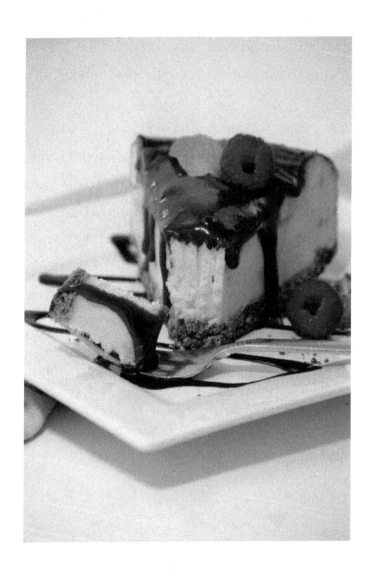

Cake with Whipped Cream Icing

Preparation Time: 20 minutes

Cooking Time: 25 minutes

Servings: 7

Ingredients:

- ¾ Cup Coconut flour

- ¾ Cup of Swerve Sweetener

- ½ Cup of Cocoa powder

- 2 Teaspoons of Baking powder

- 6 Large Eggs

- 2/3 Cup of Heavy Whipping Cream

- ½ Cup of Melted almond Butter

For whipped Cream Icing:

- 1 Cup of Heavy Whipping Cream

- ¼ Cup of Swerve Sweetener

- 1 Teaspoon of Vanilla extract

- 1/3 Cup of Sifted Cocoa Powder

Directions:

1.Pre-heat your oven to a temperature of about 350 F.

2.Grease an 8x8 cake tray with cooking spray.

3.Add the coconut flour, the Swerve sweetener; the cocoa powder, the baking powder, the eggs, the melted butter; and combine very well with an electric or a hand mixer.

4.Pour your batter into the cake tray and bake for about 25 minutes.

5.Remove the cake tray from the oven and let cool for about 5 minutes.

For the Icing

6.Whip the cream until it becomes fluffy; then add in the Swerve, the vanilla and the cocoa powder.

7.Add the Swerve, the vanilla and the cocoa powder; then continue mixing until your ingredients are very well combined.

8.Frost your baked cake with the icing!

Nutrition

357 Calories

11g Carbohydrates

2g Fiber

Walnut-Fruit Cake

Preparation Time: 15 minutes

Cooking Time: 20 minutes

Servings: 7

Ingredients:

- 1/2 Cup of almond butter (softened)
- ¼ Cup of so Nourished granulated erythritol
- 1 Tablespoon of ground cinnamon
- ½ Teaspoon of ground nutmeg
- ¼ Teaspoon of ground cloves
- 4 Large pastured eggs
- 1 Teaspoon of vanilla extract
- ½ Teaspoon of almond extract
- 2 Cups of almond flour
- ½ Cup of chopped walnuts
- ¼ Cup of dried of unsweetened cranberries
- ¼ Cup of seedless raisins

Directions:

1.Preheat your oven to a temperature of about 350 F and grease an 8-inch baking tin of round shape with coconut oil.

2.Beat the granulated erythritol on a high speed until it becomes fluffy.

3.Add the cinnamon, the nutmeg, and the cloves; then blend your ingredients until they become smooth.

4.Crack in the eggs and beat very well by adding one at a time, plus the almond extract and the vanilla.

5.Whisk in the almond flour until it forms a smooth batter then fold in the nuts and the fruit.

6.Spread your mixture into your prepared baking pan and bake it for about 20 minutes.

7.Remove the cake from the oven and let cool for about 5 minutes.

8.Dust the cake with the powdered erythritol.

Nutrition

250 Calories

12g Carbohydrates

2g Fiber

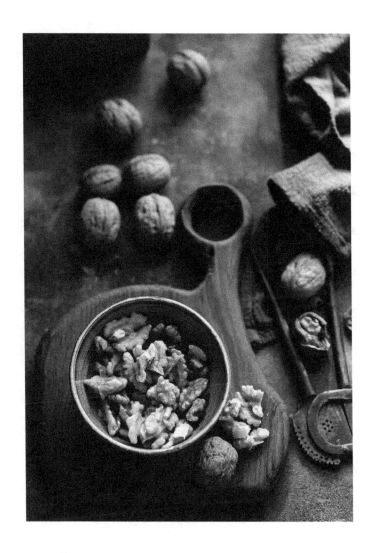

Ginger Cake

Preparation Time: 15 minutes

Cooking Time: 20 minutes

Servings: 9

Ingredients:

- ½ Tablespoon of unsalted almond butter to grease the pan

- 4 Large eggs

- ¼ Cup coconut milk

- 2 Tablespoons of unsalted almond butter

- 1 and ½ teaspoons of stevia

- 1 Tablespoon of ground cinnamon

- 1 Tablespoon of natural cocoa powder

- 1 Tablespoon of fresh ground ginger

- ½ Teaspoon of kosher salt

- 1 and ½ cups of blanched almond flour

- ½ Teaspoon of baking soda

Directions:

1.Preheat your oven to a temperature of 325 F.

2.Grease a glass baking tray of about 8X8 inches generously with almond butter.

3.In a large bowl, whisk all together the coconut milk, the eggs, the melted almond butter, the stevia, the cinnamon, the cocoa powder, the ginger and the kosher salt.

4.Whisk in the almond flour, then the baking soda and mix very well.

5.Pour the batter into the prepared pan and bake for about 20 to 25 minutes.

6.Let the cake cool for about 5 minutes.

Nutrition

175 Calories

5g Carbohydrates

1.9g Fiber

Orange Cake

Preparation Time: 10 minutes

Cooking Time: 50minutes

Servings: 8

Ingredients:

- 2 and ½ cups of almond flour

- 2 Unwaxed washed oranges

- 5 Large separated eggs

- 1 Teaspoon of baking powder

- 2 Teaspoons of orange extract

- 1 Teaspoon of vanilla bean powder

- 6 Seeds of cardamom pods crushed

- 16 drops of liquid stevia; about 3 teaspoons

- 1 Handful of flaked almonds to decorate

Directions:

1.Preheat your oven to a temperature of about 350 Fahrenheit.

2.Line a rectangular bread baking tray with a parchment paper.

3.Place the oranges into a pan filled with cold water and cover it with a lid.

4.Bring the saucepan to a boil, then let simmer for about 1 hour and make sure the oranges are totally submerged.

5.Make sure the oranges are always submerged to remove any taste of bitterness.

6.Cut the oranges into halves; then remove any seeds; and drain the water and set the oranges aside to cool down.

7.Cut the oranges in half and remove any seeds, then puree it with a blender or a food processor.

8.Separate the eggs; then whisk the egg whites until you see stiff peaks forming.

9.Add all your ingredients except for the egg whites to the orange mixture and add in the egg whites; then mix.

10.Pour the batter into the cake tin and sprinkle with the flaked almonds right on top.

11.Bake your cake for about 50 minutes.

12.Remove the cake from the oven and set aside to cool for 5 minutes.

Nutrition

164 Calories

7.1g Carbohydrates

2.7g Fiber

Lemon Cake

Preparation Time: 20 minutes

Cooking Time: 20minutes

Servings: 9

Ingredients:

- 2 Medium lemons

- 4 Large eggs

- 2 Tablespoons of almond butter

- 2 Tablespoons of avocado oil

- 1/3 cup of coconut flour

- 4-5 tablespoons of honey (or another sweetener of your choice)

- ½ tablespoon of baking soda

Directions:

1.Preheat your oven to a temperature of about 350 F.

2.Crack the eggs in a large bowl and set two egg whites aside.

3.Whisk the 2 whites of eggs with the egg yolks, the honey, the oil, the almond butter, the lemon zest and the juice and whisk very well together.

4.Combine the baking soda with the coconut flour and gradually add this dry mixture to the wet ingredients and keep whisking for a couple of minutes.

5.Beat the two eggs with a hand mixer and beat the egg into foam.

6.Add the white egg foam gradually to the mixture with a silicone spatula.

7.Transfer your obtained batter to tray covered with a baking paper.

8.Bake your cake for about 20 to 22 minutes.

9.Let the cake cool for 5 minutes; then slice your cake.

Nutrition

164 Calories

7.1g Carbohydrates

2.7g Fiber

Cinnamon Cake

Preparation Time: 15 minutes

Cooking Time: 35minutes

Servings: 8

Ingredients

For Cinnamon Filling:

- 3 Tablespoons of Swerve Sweetener

- 2 Teaspoons of ground cinnamon

For the Cake:

- 3 Cups of almond flour

- ¾ Cup of Swerve Sweetener

- ¼ Cup of unflavored whey protein powder

- 2 Teaspoon of baking powder

- ½ Teaspoon of salt

- 3 large pastured eggs

- ½ Cup of melted coconut oil

- ½ Teaspoon of vanilla extract

- ½ Cup of almond milk

- 1 Tablespoon of melted coconut oil

For cream cheese Frosting:

- 3 Tablespoons of softened cream cheese

- 2 Tablespoons of powdered Swerve Sweetener

- 1 Tablespoon of coconut heavy whipping cream

- ½ Teaspoon of vanilla extract

Directions:

1.Preheat your oven to a temperature of about 325 F and grease a baking tray of 8x8 inch.

2.For the filling, mix the Swerve and the cinnamon in a mixing bowl and mix very well; then set it aside.

3.For the preparation of the cake; whisk all together the almond flour, the sweetener, the protein powder, the baking powder, and the salt in a mixing bowl.

4.Add in the eggs, the melted coconut oil and the vanilla extract and mix very well.

5.Add in the almond milk and keep stirring until your ingredients are very well combined.

6.Spread about half of the batter in the prepared pan; then sprinkle with about two thirds of the filling mixture.

7.Spread the remaining mixture of the batter over the filling and smooth it with a spatula.

8.Bake for about 35 minutes in the oven.

9.Brush with the melted coconut oil and sprinkle with the remaining cinnamon filling.

10.Prepare the frosting by beating the cream cheese, the powdered erythritol, the cream and the vanilla extract in a mixing bowl until it becomes smooth.

11.Drizzle frost over the cooled cake.

Nutrition

222 Calories

5.4g Carbohydrates

1.5g Fiber

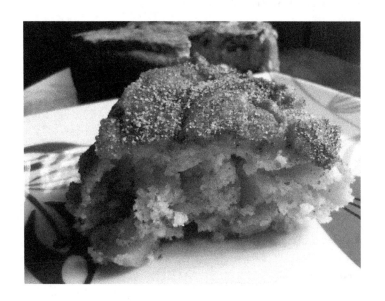

Madeleine

Preparation Time: 10 minutes

Cooking Time: 15 minutes

Servings: 12

Ingredients

- 2 Large pastured eggs

- ¾ Cup of almond flour

- 1 and ½ Tablespoons of Swerve

- ¼ Cup of cooled, melted coconut oil

- 1 Teaspoon of vanilla extract

- 1 Teaspoon of almond extract

- 1 Teaspoon of lemon zest

- ¼ Teaspoon of salt

Directions

1.Preheat your oven to a temperature of about 350 F.

2.Combine the eggs with the salt and whisk on a high speed for about 5 minutes.

3.Slowly add in the Swerve and keep mixing on high for 2 additional minutes.

4.Stir in the almond flour until it is very well-incorporated; then add in the vanilla and the almond extracts.

5.Add in the melted coconut oil and stir all your ingredients together.

6.Pour the obtained batter into equal parts in a greased Madeleine tray.

7.Bake your Ketogenic Madeleine for about 13 minutes or until the edges start to have a brown color.

8.Flip the Madeleines out of the baking tray.

Nutrition

87 Calories

3g Carbohydrates

3g Fiber

Waffles

Preparation Time: 20 minutes

Cooking Time: 30 minutes

Servings: 3

Ingredients:

For Ketogenic waffles:

- 8 Oz of cream cheese

- 5 Large pastured eggs

- 1/3 Cup of coconut flour

- ½ Teaspoon of Xanthan gum

- 1 Pinch of salt

- ½ Teaspoon of vanilla extract

- 2 Tablespoons of Swerve

- ¼ Teaspoon of baking soda

- 1/3 Cup of almond milk

Optional ingredients:

- ½ Teaspoon of cinnamon pie spice

- ¼ Teaspoon of almond extract

For low-carb Maple Syrup:

- 1 Cup of water

- 1 Tablespoon of Maple flavor

- ¾ Cup of powdered Swerve

- 1 Tablespoon of almond butter

- ½ Teaspoon of Xanthan gum

Directions

For the waffles:

1.Make sure all your ingredients are exactly at room temperature.

2.Place all your ingredients for the waffles from cream cheese to pastured eggs, coconut flour, Xanthan gum, salt, vanilla extract, the Swerve, the baking soda and the almond milk except for the almond milk with the help of a processor.

3.Blend your ingredients until it becomes smooth and creamy; then transfer the batter to a bowl.

4.Add the almond milk and mix your ingredients with a spatula.

5.Heat a waffle maker to a temperature of high.

6.Spray your waffle maker with coconut oil and add about ¼ of the batter in it evenly with a spatula into your waffle iron.

7.Close your waffle and cook until you get the color you want.

8.Carefully remove the waffles to a platter.

For the Ketogenic Maple Syrup:

9.Place 1 and ¼ cups of water, the swerve and the maple in a small pan and bring to a boil over a low heat; then let simmer for about 10 minutes.

10.Add the coconut oil.

11.Sprinkle the Xanthan gum over the top of the waffle and use an immersion blender to blend smoothly.

12.Serve and enjoy your delicious waffles!

Nutrition

316 Calories

7g Carbohydrates

3g Fiber

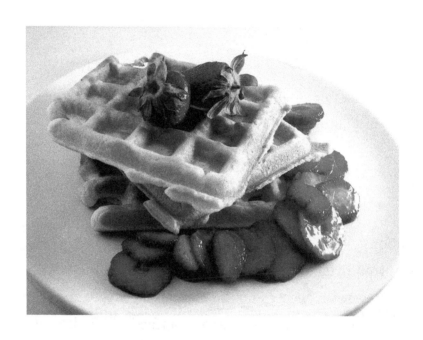

Pretzels

Preparation Time: 10 minutes

Cooking Time: 20 minutes

Servings: 8

Ingredients:

- 1 and ½ cups of pre-shredded mozzarella

- 2 Tablespoons of full fat cream cheese

- 1 Large egg

- ¾ Cup of almond flour+ 2 tablespoons of ground almonds or almond meal

- ½ Teaspoon of baking powder

- 1 Pinch of coarse sea salt

Directions:

1.Heat your oven to a temperature of about 180 C/356 F.

2.Melt the cream cheese and the mozzarella cheese and stir over a low heat until the cheeses are perfectly melted.

3.If you choose to microwave the cheese, just do that for about 1 minute no more and if you want to do it on the stove, turn off the heat as soon as the cheese is completely melted.

4.Add the large egg to the prepared warm dough; then stir until your ingredients are very well combined. If the egg is cold; you will need to heat it gently.

5.Add in the ground almonds or the almond flour and the baking powder and stir until your ingredients are very well combined.

6.Take one pinch of the dough of cheese and toll it or stretch it in your hands until it is about 18 to 20 cm of length; if your dough is sticky, you can oil your hands to avoid that.

7.Now, form pretzels from the cheese dough and nicely shape it; then place it over a baking sheet.

8.Sprinkle with a little bit of salt and bake for about 17 minutes.

Nutrition

113 Calories

2.5g Carbohydrates

0.8g Fiber

Cheesy Taco Bites

Preparation Time: 5 minutes

Cooking Time: 10minutes

Serving: 12

Ingredients

- 2 Cups of Packaged Shredded Cheddar Cheese

- 2 Tablespoon of Chili Powder

- 2 Tablespoons of Cumin

- 1 Teaspoon of Salt

- 8 Teaspoons of coconut cream for garnishing

- Use Pico de Gallo for garnishing as well

Directions:

1.Preheat your oven to a temperature of about 350 F.

2.Over a baking sheet lined with a parchment paper, place 1 tablespoon piles of cheese and make sure to a space of 2 inches between each.

3.Place the baking sheet in your oven and bake for about 5 minutes.

4.Remove from the oven and let the cheese cool down for about 1 minute; then carefully lift up and press each into the cups of a mini muffin tin.

5.Make sure to press the edges of the cheese to form the shape of muffins mini.

6.Let the cheese cool completely; then remove it.

7.While you continue to bake the cheese and create your cups.

8.Fill the cheese cups with the coconut cream, then top with the Pico de Gallo.

Nutrition

73 Calories

3g Carbohydrates

4g Protein

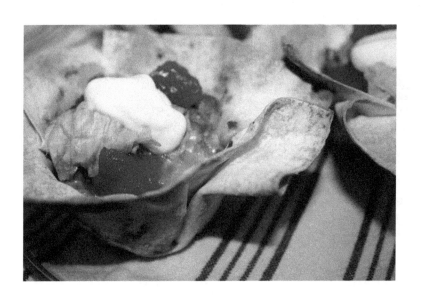

Nut Squares

Preparation Time: 30 minutes

Cooking Time: 10 minutes

Serving: 10

Ingredients:

- 2 Cups of almonds, pumpkin seeds, sunflower seeds and walnuts

- ½ Cup of desiccated coconut

- 1 Tablespoon of chia seeds

- ¼ Teaspoon of salt

- 2 Tablespoons of coconut oil

- 1 Teaspoon of vanilla extract

- 3 Tablespoons of almond or peanut butter

- 1/3 Cup of Sukrin Gold Fiber Syrup

Directions:

1.Line a square baking tin with a baking paper; then lightly grease it with cooking spray

2.Chop all the nuts roughly; then slightly grease it too, you can also leave them as whole

3.Mix the nuts in a large bowl; then combine them in a large bowl with the coconut, the chia seeds and the salt

4.In a microwave-proof bowl; add the coconut oil; then add the vanilla, the coconut butter or oil, the almond butter and the fiber syrup and microwave the mixture for about 30 seconds

5.Stir your ingredients together very well; then pour the melted mixture right on top of the nuts

6.Press the mixture into your prepared baking tin with the help of the back of a measuring cup and push very well

7.Freeze your treat for about 1 hour before cutting it

8.Cut your frozen nut batter into small cubes or squares of the same size

Nutrition

268 Calories

14g Carbohydrates

1g Fiber

Smoothies

Blueberry Smoothie

Preparation Time: 10 minutes

Cooking Time: 0 minutes

Servings: 2

Ingredients:

- 2 cups frozen blueberries

- 1 small banana

- 1½ cups unsweetened almond milk

- ¼ cup ice cubes

Directions:

1. Place all the ingredients in a high-speed blender and pulse until creamy.

2. Pour the smoothie into two glasses and serve immediately.

Nutrition: Calories 158 Total Fat 3.3 g Saturated Fat 0.3 g Cholesterol 0 mg Sodium 137 mg Total Carbs 34 g Fiber 5.6 g Sugar 20.6 g Protein 2.4 g

Beet & Strawberry Smoothie

Preparation Time: 10 minutes

Cooking Time: 0 minutes

Servings: 2

Ingredients:

- 2 cups frozen strawberries, pitted and chopped

- 2/3 cup roasted and frozen beet, chopped

- 1 teaspoon fresh ginger, peeled and grated

- 1 teaspoon fresh turmeric, peeled and grated

- ½ cup fresh orange juice

- 1 cup unsweetened almond milk

Directions:

1. Place all the ingredients in a high-speed blender and pulse until creamy.

2. Pour the smoothie into two glasses and serve immediately.

Nutrition: Calories 258 Total Fat 1.5 g Saturated Fat 0.1 g Cholesterol 0 mg Sodium 134 mg Total Carbs 26.7g Fiber 4.9 g Sugar 18.7 g Protein 2.9 g

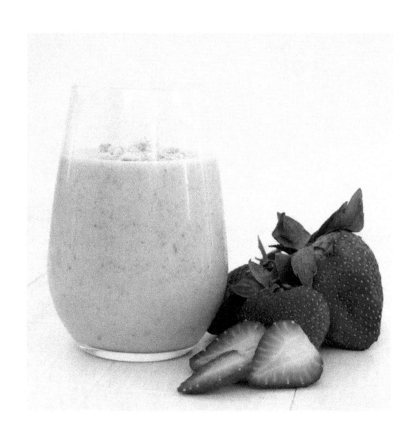

Kiwi Smoothie

Preparation Time: 10 minutes
Cooking Time: 0 minutes
Servings: 2
Ingredients:

- 4 kiwis

- 2 small bananas, peeled

- 1½ cups unsweetened almond milk

- 1-2 drops liquid stevia

- ¼ cup ice cubes

Directions:

1. Place all the ingredients in a high-speed blender and pulse until creamy.

2. Pour the smoothie into two glasses and serve immediately.

Nutrition: Calories 228 Total Fat 3.8 g Saturated Fat 0.4 g Cholesterol 0 mg Sodium 141 mg Total Carbs 50.7 g Fiber 8.4 g Sugar 28.1 g Protein 3.8 g

Pineapple & Carrot Smoothie

Preparation Time: 10 minutes
Cooking Time: 0 minutes
Servings: 2
Ingredients:

- 1 cup frozen pineapple

- 1 large ripe banana, peeled and sliced

- ½ tablespoon fresh ginger, peeled and chopped

- ¼ teaspoon ground turmeric

- 1 cup unsweetened almond milk

- ½ cup fresh carrot juice

- 1 tablespoon fresh lemon juice

Directions:

1. Place all the ingredients in a high-speed blender and pulse until creamy.

2. Pour the smoothie into two glasses and serve immediately.

Nutrition: Calories 132 Total Fat 2.2 g Saturated Fat 0.3 g Cholesterol 0 mg Sodium 113 mg Total Carbs 629.3 g Fiber 4.1 g Sugar 16.9 g Protein 2 g

Oats & Orange Smoothie

Preparation Time: 10 minutes
Cooking Time: 0 minutes
Servings: 4
Ingredients:

- 2/3 cup rolled oats

- 2 oranges, peeled, seeded, and sectioned

- 2 large bananas, peeled and sliced

- 2 cups unsweetened almond milk

- 1 cup ice cubes, crushed

Directions:

1. Place all the ingredients in a high-speed blender and pulse until creamy.

2. Pour the smoothie into four glasses and serve immediately.

Nutrition: Calories 175

Total Fat 3 g Saturated Fat 0.4 g Cholesterol 0 mg Sodium 93 mg Total Carbs 36.6 g Fiber 5.9 g Sugar 17.1 g Protein 3.9 g

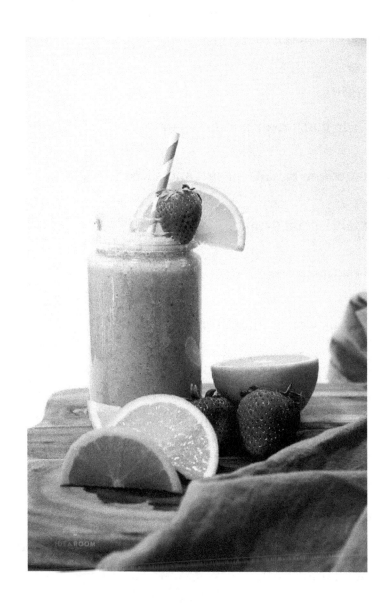

Pumpkin Smoothie

Preparation Time: 10 minutes

Cooking Time: 0 minutes

Servings: 2

Ingredients:

- 1 cup homemade pumpkin puree

- 1 medium banana, peeled and sliced

- 1 tablespoon maple syrup

- 1 teaspoon ground flaxseeds

- ½ teaspoon ground cinnamon

- ¼ teaspoon ground ginger

- 1½ cups unsweetened almond milk

- ¼ cup ice cubes

Directions:

1. Place all the ingredients in a high-speed blender and pulse until creamy.

2. Pour the smoothie into two glasses and serve immediately.

Nutrition: Calories 159 Total Fat 3.6 g Saturated Fat 0.5 g Cholesterol 0 mg Sodium 143 mg Total Carbs 32.6 g Fiber 6.5 g Sugar 17.3 g Protein 3 g

Red Veggie & Fruit Smoothie

Preparation Time: 10 minutes
Cooking Time: 0 minutes
Servings: 2
Ingredients:

- ½ cup fresh raspberries

- ½ cup fresh strawberries

- ½ red bell pepper, seeded and chopped

- ½ cup red cabbage, chopped

- 1 small tomato

- 1 cup water

- ½ cup ice cubes

Directions:

1. Place all the ingredients in a high-speed blender and pulse until creamy.

2. Pour the smoothie into two glasses and serve immediately.

Nutrition: Calories 39 Cholesterol 0 mg Saturated Fat 0 g Sodium 10 mg Total Carbs 8.9 g Fiber 3.5 g Sugar 4.8 g Protein 1.3 g Total Fat 0.4 g

Kale Smoothie

Preparation Time: 10 minutes
Cooking Time: 0 minutes
Servings: 2
Ingredients:

- 3 stalks fresh kale, trimmed and chopped

- 1-2 celery stalks, chopped

- ½ avocado, peeled, pitted, and chopped

- ½-inch piece ginger root, chopped

- ½-inch piece turmeric root, chopped

- 2 cups coconut milk

Directions:

1. Place all the ingredients in a high-speed blender and pulse until creamy.

2. Pour the smoothie into two glasses and serve
   immediately.

Nutrition: Calories 248 Total Fat 21.8 g Saturated Fat 12 g
Cholesterol 0 mg Sodium 59 mg Total Carbs 11.3 g Fiber 4.2 g
Sugar 0.5 g Protein 3.5 g

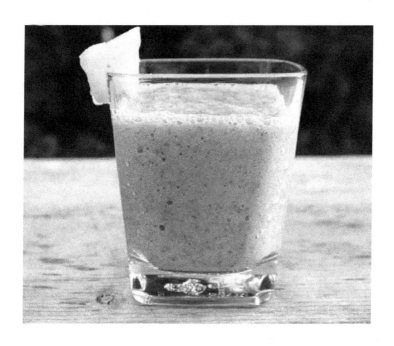

Green Tofu Smoothie

Preparation Time: 10 minutes
Cooking Time: 0 minutes
Servings: 2
Ingredients:

- 1½ cups cucumber, peeled and chopped roughly

- 3 cups fresh baby spinach

- 2 cups frozen broccoli

- ½ cup silken tofu, drained and pressed

- 1 tablespoon fresh lime juice

- 4-5 drops liquid stevia

- 1 cup unsweetened almond milk

- ½ cup ice, crushed

Directions:

1. Place all the ingredients in a high-speed blender and pulse until creamy.

2. Pour the smoothie into two glasses and serve immediately.

Nutrition: Calories 118 Total Fat 15 g Saturated Fat 0.8 g Cholesterol 0 mg Sodium 165 mg Total Carbs 12.6 g Fiber 4.8 g Sugar 3.4 g Protein 10 g

Grape & Swiss Chard Smoothie

Preparation Time: 10 minutes
Cooking Time: 0 minutes
Servings: 2
Ingredients:

- 2 cups seedless green grapes

- 2 cups fresh Swiss chard, trimmed and chopped

- 2 tablespoons maple syrup

- 1 teaspoon fresh lemon juice

- 1½ cups water

- 4 ice cubes

Directions:

1. Place all the ingredients in a high-speed blender and pulse until creamy.

2. Pour the smoothie into two glasses and serve immediately.

Nutrition: Calories 176 Total Fat 0.2 g Saturated Fat 0 g Cholesterol 0 mg Sodium 83 mg Total Carbs 44.9 g Fiber 1.7 g Sugar 37.9 g Protein 0.7 g

Matcha Smoothie

Preparation Time: 10 minutes

Cooking Time: 0 minutes

Servings: 2

Ingredients:

- 2 tablespoons chia seeds

- 2 teaspoons matcha green tea powder

- ½ teaspoon fresh lemon juice

- ½ teaspoon xanthan gum

- 8-10 drops liquid stevia

- 4 tablespoons coconut cream

- 1½ cups unsweetened almond milk

- ¼ cup ice cubes

Directions:

1. Place all the ingredients in a high-speed blender and pulse until creamy.

2. Pour the smoothie into two glasses and serve immediately.

Nutrition: Calories 132 Total Fat 12.3 g Saturated Fat 6.8 g Cholesterol 0 mg Sodium 15 mg Total Carbs 7 g Fiber 4.8 g Sugar 1 g Protein 3 g

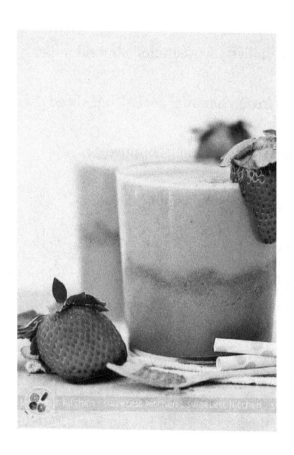

Banana Smoothie

Preparation Time: 10 minutes

Cooking Time: 0 minutes

Servings: 2

Ingredients:

- 2 cups chilled unsweetened almond milk

- 1 large frozen banana, peeled and sliced

- 1 tablespoon almonds, chopped

- 1 teaspoon organic vanilla extract

Directions:

1. Place all the ingredients in a high-speed blender and pulse until creamy.

2. Pour the smoothie into two glasses and serve immediately.

Nutrition: Calories 124 Total Fat 5.2 g Saturated Fat 0.5 g Cholesterol 0 mg Sodium 181 mg Total Carbs 18.4 g Fiber 3.1 g Sugar 8.7 g Protein 2.4 g

Strawberry Smoothie

Preparation Time: 10 minutes

Cooking Time: 0 minutes

Servings: 2

Ingredients:

- 2 cups chilled unsweetened almond milk

- 1½ cups frozen strawberries

- 1 banana, peeled and sliced

- ¼ teaspoon organic vanilla extract

Directions:

1. Add all the ingredients in a high-speed blender and pulse until smooth.

2. Pour the smoothie into two glasses and serve immediately.

Nutrition: Calories 131 Total Fat 3.7 g Saturated Fat 0.4 g Cholesterol 0 mg Sodium 181 mg Total Carbs 25.3 g Fiber 4.8 g Sugar 14 g Protein 1.6 g

CPSIA information can be obtained
at www.ICGtesting.com
Printed in the USA
BVHW010850050521
606355BV00008B/37